BABY'S FIRST FOODS

Introduction

As a first-time mom and a nurse, I've always approached parenting with a blend of curiosity, caution, and care. When it came time to introduce solids to my baby, I found myself at a crossroads. The traditional recommendations—starting solids at 4 months, giving purees, and introducing baby cereals—just didn't sit right with me. As a nurse, I knew there was more to the picture when it came to nutrition and development. But beyond my professional background, I have a deeply personal reason for questioning the norm: a family history of **Crohn's disease, IBS**, and other gastrointestinal issues. These conditions have affected several generations of my family, and I knew that feeding practices played a role in gut health.

The more I researched and learned about ancestral diets which are rich in nutrient-dense, whole foods, the more I realized that this was the path that aligned with both my professional knowledge and my family's unique health needs. I wanted to give my baby the very best start by focusing on foods that nourish and strengthen the gut, promote brain development, and build a foundation for long-term health.

This book is the result of that journey, a step-by-step guide to introducing **nutrient-dense, ancestral foods** to babies, in a way that feels natural, intuitive, and rooted in tradition. It's an approach that goes beyond the conventional, because I truly believe it's the best way to nourish our little ones from the very beginning.

The information presented in this book is based on my personal experience as a mother and nurse, as well as extensive research into ancestral nutrition and traditional feeding practices. It is intended for educational and informational purposes only.

This book does **not** constitute medical advice and is not a substitute for professional guidance from your pediatrician, healthcare provider, or registered dietitian. Every child is unique, and what worked well for my baby may not be appropriate for yours. Always consult with your child's healthcare provider before making any changes to their diet or feeding routine—especially if your child has known medical conditions, allergies, or developmental concerns.

The author and publisher disclaim any liability for adverse reactions or consequences resulting from the use of information contained in this book.

Welcome!

Feeding your baby is one of the most important decisions you will make as a parent. In a world filled with pre-packaged, ultra-processed baby foods and confusing nutritional advice, it can feel overwhelming to know what's truly best for your child. But what if the answers to optimal infant nutrition weren't found in modern formulas and cereals, but rather in the diets of our ancestors that are rich in whole, unprocessed, nutrient-dense foods that have nourished generations of thriving, healthy humans?

Baby's First Foods: Nourishing the Gut with Ancestral Basics is your step-by-step guide to introducing first foods that align with time-tested, traditional wisdom. The ancestral diet is rooted in real, whole foods, especially nutrient-dense animal products that provide the essential building blocks for your baby's brain, gut, and overall physical development. Unlike conventional baby foods, which often rely on refined grains, synthetic vitamins, and low-fat formulas, an ancestral approach focuses on bioavailable nutrients that babies can absorb and utilize efficiently.

For thousands of years, traditional societies introduced babies to foods that were naturally rich in essential fats, proteins, fat-soluble vitamins, and probiotics which were elements critical for a robust immune system, cognitive function, and a resilient gut microbiome. From pastured egg yolks and bone broths to organ meats and fermented foods, these nourishing staples have been largely abandoned in favor of modern, industrialized baby food products that lack the same nutritional integrity.

This book will walk you through exactly *what* to feed your baby and *why*, providing an easy-to-follow roadmap for introducing nutrient-rich, gut-friendly first foods. By going back to the basics, you'll be equipping your child with the best foundation for a lifetime of health—supporting strong bones, a well-developed nervous system, and strong immune system, all while reducing the risk of allergies, digestive issues, and metabolic disorders later in life.

If you're ready to move beyond outdated feeding guidelines and embrace a nourishing, ancestral approach to baby's first foods, this book will be your ultimate companion. Welcome to a journey of rediscovering the power of real food, the way nature intended.

Chapter One: The Health Benefits of an Ancestral Diet

The first year of your little one's life is a critical window for growth and development, both physically and neurologically. Every bite of food introduced during this time serves a purpose, shaping their brain function, gut microbiome, immune system, and long-term metabolic health. This is why choosing the *right* foods is so important.

For thousands of years, traditional cultures instinctively knew what foods best supported infant health. Across the world, babies were weaned onto nutrient-rich animal products, bone broths, and fermented foods long before modern science confirmed their benefits.

For example:

- Indigenous Arctic populations introduced fish roe, organ meats, and seal blubber as first foods.

- Traditional African diets included iron-rich meats, bone broths, and fermented porridge.

- Asian cultures have long used miso, natto, and broth-based soups to support digestion and immunity.

In today's world, processed baby foods and fortified cereals are marketed as the best options for first foods. However, these products often lack the nutrient density and bioavailability necessary for optimal development. In contrast, an ancestral diet, one based on the nutrient-dense, whole foods our ancestors relied on provides the most complete nourishment for growing babies.

These traditions existed because they worked by producing strong, resilient children without the chronic health issues so common today. By returning to this wisdom, we are reconnecting with a way of feeding that has sustained humanity for generations.

Let's dive into the core benefits of this traditional way of eating and why it gives your child the best foundation for a lifetime of health.

1. Born to Eat This Way: It's Physiological

An ancestral diet prioritizes foods that are naturally *rich* in vitamins, minerals, healthy fats, and proteins. Remember, unlike fortified foods that use synthetic nutrients, ancestral foods provide **bioavailable** nutrition, meaning the body can absorb and utilize them effectively.

Babies are born with **digestive enzymes** best suited for breaking down fats and proteins from animal sources— its purely physiological:

- **Lipase** (found in breastmilk) helps digest fats from butter, egg yolks, and animal fats. This makes sense why breastmilk is the first food and is high in fat - particularly saturated fat and cholesterol which are vital for brain development.

- **Protease** breaks down proteins like those in meat, fish, and dairy.

- **Amylase**, the enzyme that digests carbohydrates, is **very low in babies under 1 year old**, making grains and starches harder to digest.

2. Brain Development: Fueling Intelligence and Cognitive Growth

The first two years of life are when the brain develops *most* rapidly, forming the neural connections that will shape intelligence, memory, and cognitive function. This requires an abundance of the right nutrients, particularly:

- **DHA (Docosahexaenoic Acid)** – A critical omega-3 fatty acid found in fatty fish, egg yolks, and grass-fed dairy. DHA is a primary structural component of the brain and retina, essential for learning and vision. More importantly, DHA promotes memory, problem solving, and learning as well as emotional regulation and mood stability.

- **Choline** – Found in egg yolks, liver, and meat, choline is vital for neurotransmitter function and memory formation.

- **B Vitamins** – Needed for energy production, mood regulation, and nervous system development. B12, found in animal foods, is particularly essential.

-
- **Foods high in fats** – there is no limit on fat consumption under 2 years old and it is needed to create myelin sheath for fast communication within brain cells. Babies who do not get enough fats in their diet may be at risk for developmental delays, mood disorders, and learning difficulties.
- Fat soluble vitamins –
    - Vitamin A is needed for brain, vision, and immune development.
    - Vitamin D is needed for brain function, bone growth, and immune regulation.
    - Vitamin E is needed to protect the brain cells from oxidative stress

- Vitamin K2 is needed for brain development and cardiovascular health

Babies who receive adequate amounts of these brain-boosting nutrients have been shown to have better cognitive function, emotional regulation, and even improved academic performance later in life.

3. Gut Health: The Foundation of a Strong Immune System

A baby's gut is still developing in the first year, and the foods they consume will play a major role in shaping their microbiome, the trillions of bacteria that influence digestion, immunity, and even mental health.

An ancestral diet supports gut health by including:

- **Bone broth, meat stock, and collagen-rich foods** – These help seal and strengthen the gut lining, preventing leaky gut and food sensitivities.

- **Fermented foods (sauerkraut, sour dough, kefir, yogurt, miso, etc.)** – Natural probiotics that promote a healthy, diverse gut microbiome.

- **Prebiotic-rich vegetables** – These feed beneficial bacteria and enhance digestion.

In contrast, modern baby foods, especially processed grains and sugars, can disrupt the gut microbiome, leading to inflammation, food allergies, and even behavioral issues as children grow. Increased sugar intake in babies can develop unhealthy taste preferences making it more challenging to introduce the savory and nutrient dense flavors of real foods. If your little one has high sugar intake, this also poses a risk at blood sugar spikes and insulin responses which can lead to metabolic issues down the road resulting in long term issues such as type 2 diabetes. It doesn't just stop there, your little one can be at risk of dental issues, prone to infections, and a potential contribution to childhood obesity.

4. Immune Support: Strengthening Defenses Naturally

A strong immune system begins with the *right* nutrition. Ancestral diets provide critical immune-boosting nutrients such as:

- **Vitamin A (from liver, egg yolks, and butter)** – Essential for immune function and fighting infections.

- **Zinc (found in chicken stock, meat, and beans)** – A mineral that helps white blood cells combat illness.

- **Vitamin D (from fatty fish, egg yolks, and sunlight)** – Regulates the immune response and protects against autoimmune diseases.

By introducing these foods early, your little one will build stronger immune resilience, reducing the likelihood of chronic illnesses, allergies, and autoimmune conditions later in life.

Setting Your Baby Up for a Lifetime of Health

By choosing an ancestral diet, you are doing more than just feeding your baby, you are laying the foundation for a lifetime of ideal health. With the right nutrition, your child will benefit from:

- Strong brain development and cognitive function
- A well-balanced gut microbiome for better digestion and immunity
- Reduced risk of allergies, autoimmune diseases, and chronic conditions
- Steady energy and blood sugar balance
- A deep connection to real, wholesome foods

This book will guide you step by step in implementing this nutrient-dense, gut-supporting approach helping you nourish your baby in the most natural and effective way possible.

The journey to lifelong health starts with what's on your baby's plate. Let's make every bite count.

Chapter Two: When to Start Solids Laying the Foundation for Lifelong Health

Is your little one ready? Starting solids is one of the most exciting milestones in your baby's first year of life. But with so much conflicting advice, many parents are left wondering: *When is the right time?* In a world where baby food companies push early introduction and outdated guidelines once recommended rice cereal as a first food, it's more important than ever to return to traditional culture and the science of infant nutrition.

The Traditional Approach to First Foods

Many traditional cultures introduced solid foods in a gradual, intentional way—starting with small amounts of nutrient-dense foods that complemented, rather than replaced, breastmilk or formula. This approach ensured babies received optimal nutrition without overwhelming their delicate digestive systems.

Instead of beginning with starch-heavy cereals, ultra processed foods, or prepackaged foods, ancestral diets prioritized:

- **Iron-rich foods** like liver, marrow, and meat
- **Healthy fats** from egg yolks, grass-fed butter, and fatty cuts of meat
- **Broths, meat stock, and fermented foods**

These foods were carefully chosen because they provided bioavailable nutrients in a form that tiny bodies could easily absorb and utilize. Keep in mind these are not man-made vegetable fats or oils. These are whole foods that provide micronutrients as building blocks down to the cellular level of your growing little one.

The Right Time: Why Waiting Until 6 Months Matters

Research and ancestral practices align on one fundamental truth, waiting until around 6 months to introduce solid foods is most beneficial for your baby's digestive system, immune health, and nutrient absorption. At birth, your baby's gut is still developing, and introducing foods too early can increase the risk of food sensitivities, digestive distress, and even allergies.

By 6 months, the gut lining has matured enough to better handle more complex foods, reducing the likelihood of leaky gut syndrome, food-related immune reactions, and disorders such as obesity down the road. Additionally, breastmilk or formula remains the primary source of nutrition in the first year, with solid foods complementing—not replacing—this foundational nourishment.

Another key factor? Around the 6-month mark, your baby's natural iron stores, inherited from the womb, begin to deplete. This is why it is critical to introduce *nutrient-dense*, iron-rich foods—not processed cereals, but real, bioavailable sources such as pastured egg yolks, liver, and bone broths. These ancestral foods provide the essential building blocks for brain development, immunity, and gut health in a way no fortified grain product ever could.

Fortified baby cereals and synthetic vitamins may seem like an easy solution for meeting a baby's nutritional needs, but they are not the most optimal choice when it comes to nourishing a developing infant, here's why:

- Your baby produces very small amounts of the enzyme that breaks down carbohydrates. This means that breaking down certain foods is challenging on your little ones digestion.
- There is a lack of nutrient density in these foods. Your little ones' rapidly developing digestive system needs food that is bioavailable, meaning

they enter the body and work right away with an active effect- like zinc, healthy fats, iron, omegas, B vitamins, fat-soluble vitamins, calcium, DHA, fiber, etc.
- Fortified foods lack beneficial compounds such as choline, collagen, and fats which are essential for brain development, gut health, and overall growth. Foods with collagen support gut lining, reduce inflammation, promote microbiome, and improve digestion.
- Foods fortified with iron are thought to supplement babies after 6 months, but iron added to fortified cereals is usually in the form of inorganic iron, which is harder for babies to digest and absorb. When the body does not process synthetic nutrients the same way we do with whole foods, this can lead to imbalances and deficiencies.
- Refined grains in baby cereals can place unnecessary strain on their immature digestive system by leading to gut inflammation. They can also contain gluten or soy which can trigger allergic reactions or sensitivities in your little one.

Signs That Your Baby is Ready

Rather than following an arbitrary timeline, the best way to know when to introduce solids is by watching for developmental cues. Your baby is likely ready if they:

- Can sit up unassisted and hold their head steady

- Show interest in food. This can be watching you eat, or reaching for your plate

- Have lost the tongue-thrust reflex (which pushes foreign objects out of the mouth)

- Can bring objects or hands to their mouth

- Still seem hungry after regular breastmilk or formula feedings

If your baby is showing these signs, their body is giving you the green light to start introducing nourishing, whole foods.

Why Breastmilk or Formula Remains Essential

A common misconception is that once solids are introduced, they should become the primary food source. However, breastmilk or formula should remain the nutritional foundation throughout the first year and beyond. Solids are meant to *complement* not replace this critical nourishment.

Why? Because breastmilk and properly formulated formulas contain:

- **Essential antibodies** to continue supporting the immune system

- **Easily digestible fats and proteins** for energy and brain development

- **Balanced nutrition** that adapts to your baby's needs, ensuring they don't miss vital nutrients during the transition to solids

Abruptly replacing milk with solid foods too soon can lead to nutritional gaps, digestive distress, and even failure to thrive. Instead, introducing solids should be a gradual process by offering nutrient-dense foods as a secondary modality while still allowing your baby to nurse or take a bottle as needed.

Chapter Three: The Building Blocks of Development

When it comes to nourishing your baby for optimal growth, not all foods are created equal. Some provide essential, bioavailable nutrients that fuel brain development, gut integrity, and immune function, while others offer little more than empty calories.

In modern feeding recommendations, parents are often told to introduce fruits, rice cereals, and vegetables early on. However, ancestral wisdom and modern research suggests that prioritizing nutrient-dense *animal-based foods* first can give your baby a significant advantage. These foods supply critical building blocks that plant-based foods simply can't match.

This chapter will explore the essential first foods that provide the *most* nourishment for your baby's growing body, explaining why they matter and how they support digestion, development, and long-term health.

1. Bone Marrow: The Ultimate Brain Food

Bone marrow is one of the most nutrient-dense superfoods on the planet, uniquely designed to support brain growth and immune function. It is packed with:

- **Healthy fats** – Critical for brain myelination (the process that helps neurons communicate efficiently).

- **Collagen and gelatin** – Essential for gut lining integrity and reducing inflammation.

- **Glycine and proline** – Amino acids that promote digestion and tissue repair.

- **Iron, zinc, and vitamin A** – Key for immune strength and neurological development.

Since bone marrow is naturally soft and buttery, it is an ideal first food for babies. It can be served straight from a roasted bone or blended into purees and broths.

2. Bone Broth & Chicken Stock: Gut-Healing Foundations

Bone broth and chicken stock are *true* foundational foods, deeply nourishing for digestion, immunity, and connective tissue development. These broths contain:

- **Gelatin and collagen** – Repair and strengthen the gut lining, crucial for preventing leaky gut and food sensitivities.

- **Glycine** – An amino acid that supports digestion, liver detoxification, and restful sleep.

- **Minerals (calcium, magnesium, phosphorus, potassium)** – Essential for bone development and nervous system regulation.

Babies are born with immature digestive systems, making gut-friendly foods like bone broth crucial for reducing inflammation and aiding nutrient absorption. A spoonful of warm broth daily can help fortify your baby's microbiome and overall resilience. I have taught my little one to drink warm chicken stock from an open faced cup with meals.

3. Butter & Animal Fats: The Fuel for Growth

For decades, fat was unfairly demonized, but ancestral diets have always recognized its vital role in child development. Babies *need* high-quality fats for energy, hormone production, and cellular function. The best sources include:

- **Grass-fed butter** – Rich in fat-soluble vitamins A, D, E, and K, which are essential for immune and bone health.

- **Tallow (beef fat) & lard (pork fat)** – Provide cholesterol, a key component for brain function and hormone production.

- **Duck fat** – High in monounsaturated fats and vitamin K2, crucial for calcium regulation and cardiovascular health.

These fats are more easily digested and utilized than plant-based oils, making them the *best* source of fuel for developing babies. They also support the absorption of fat-soluble vitamins from other foods.

4. Egg Yolks: Nature's Perfect Baby Food

Egg yolks are one of the most complete foods a baby can consume, containing nearly every nutrient needed for development. They are especially rich in:

- **Choline** – Essential for brain development and neurotransmitter function.

- **DHA & EPA (Omega-3s)** – Critical for vision, cognitive function, and reducing inflammation.

- **Biotin & B vitamins** – Support energy production and metabolism.

- **Vitamin A & D** – Strengthen immunity and skeletal development.

Unlike egg whites, which contain anti-nutrients that may be harder for infants to digest, egg yolks are gentle on the gut and can be introduced early preferably from pastured eggs for the highest nutrient content. Make sure they are cooked all the way properly.

5. Organ Meats: Nature's Multivitamin

Liver, heart, and other organ meats are *far* more nutrient-dense than muscle meats alone, making them an essential part of an ancestral baby diet. Liver, in particular, is one of the best first foods for babies due to its unmatched concentration of:

- **Iron** – Highly bioavailable heme iron prevents anemia and supports red blood cell production.

- **Vitamin A** – Crucial for vision, immune defense, and cellular growth.

- **B Vitamins (B12, B6, Folate, Riboflavin)** – Support energy, brain function, and DNA synthesis.

- **Copper & Zinc** – Essential for immune function and metabolic processes.

A small amount of pureed liver (from grass-fed or pasture-raised sources) once or twice a week can provide an incredible boost to your baby's nutrient intake. Little amounts can be added onto a slice of sourdough but you want to make sure you don't overdo it as you little one can be susceptible to vitamin A toxicity.

6. Beef & Other Ruminant Meats: The Best Source of Iron & Protein

Beef, lamb, and other ruminant meats are among the most nourishing foods for babies, particularly because they offer:

- **Heme iron** – Easily absorbed, preventing iron deficiency as baby's stores deplete around 6 months.

- **High-quality protein** – Needed for muscle development, enzyme production, and tissue repair.

- **Zinc** – Vital for immune function, growth, and digestion.

Compared to chicken or pork, beef and lamb provide higher levels of essential fatty acids and fat-soluble vitamins, making them superior choices for a baby's first meats.

Why Hold Off on Fruit?

While fruits are often one of the first foods introduced to babies, there are reasons to delay their introduction in favor of more nutrient-dense options:

- **Sugar content** – Even natural fruit sugars can alter taste preferences early on, leading to a preference for sweet foods over nutrient-rich savory options.

- **Sorbitol content** - Can impact the absorption of nutrients from other foods.

- **Lack of essential fats & proteins** – Fruits do not provide the critical building blocks needed for brain and gut development.

This doesn't mean fruit should be *completely* avoided—just that it should come *after* nutrient-dense animal foods have been established. When introduced later, berries and low-glycemic fruits are good options.

Chapter Four: A Step-by-Step Guide to Starting Solids

Now that you understand why an ancestral diet is the most nourishing way to introduce solids, let's break down exactly *how* to begin. Many parents feel overwhelmed when it comes to transitioning their baby to real food, but it doesn't have to be complicated.

By following a structured, gradual approach, you can help your baby's digestion adjust smoothly while ensuring they receive the most nutrient-dense foods right from the start.

This chapter outlines a **7-step plan** to introduce ancestral first foods in a way that supports gut health, brain development, and metabolic balance. First we will begin with highlighting different options for introducing foods to your little one. You can begin with purees or start right away with baby led weaning:

How to Start Baby-Led Weaning (BLW) at 6 Months with an Ancestral Diet

Baby-Led Weaning (BLW) is a **natural approach to introducing solids**, allowing babies to explore whole foods in their original form rather than spoon-fed purees.

When paired with an **ancestral diet**, BLW becomes an excellent way to support **gut health, brain development, and immune function** while honoring traditional wisdom.

Step 1: Preparing for BLW

Before starting, make sure:

🦴 Your baby is **6 months old** and showing signs of readiness.
🦴 Your baby has **good head and neck control** and can sit upright with support.
🦴 You understand **safe food textures** and how to modify foods to reduce choking risk.
🦴 Your baby is still **breastfeeding or formula feeding**, as solids complement but do not replace milk at this stage.

Step 2: First Foods – Prioritizing Nutrient-Dense Options

An ancestral approach to BLW focuses on **fat-rich, bioavailable, and gut-friendly** foods first, rather than grains or starches.

Best First Foods for BLW (6-7 Months)

🫘 **Animal-Based Nutrient Powerhouses:**

- **Bone marrow** (soft, scoopable, rich in healthy fats)

- **Bone broth or chicken stock** (can be spoon-fed or used to soften foods)

- **Grass-fed butter, ghee, or tallow** (easy to digest, similar to breastmilk fats)

- **Soft-cooked egg yolk** (rich in choline for brain development)

- **Slow-cooked shredded meats** (like lamb, beef, or chicken)

- **Liver pâté** (iron and vitamin A powerhouse, serve in small amounts)

- **Sardines (with bones, mashed)** (high in omega-3s and calcium)

🥕 **Vegetables That Complement an Ancestral Diet:**
Since babies **lack the enzymes to properly digest grains and starches**, we focus on **non-starchy vegetables rich in fat-soluble vitamins**:

- **Avocado** (healthy fats, creamy texture)
- **Cooked carrots** (rich in vitamin A, serve with butter)
- **Roasted zucchini or squash** (easy to grasp and digest)
- **Steamed asparagus or green beans** (cut into finger-length pieces)
- **Cooked and buttered spinach or kale** (for iron and minerals)

💡 **Tip:** Always **serve vegetables with healthy fats** like butter, ghee, or animal fats to **enhance nutrient absorption** (especially vitamins A, D, E, and K).

Step 3: How to Serve Foods Safely

🦴 **6-7 Months:** Large, soft strips of food for baby to grab (e.g., long strips of steak, roasted squash, or soft-cooked carrots)

🦴 **8-9 Months:** Smaller pieces for improved pincer grasp (e.g., minced meats, avocado strips, cottage cheese).

🦴 **10-12 Months:** More textures and variety, allowing for self-feeding with utensils.

🛑 **Choking Prevention Tips:**

- Ensure food is **soft and easy to mash between fingers**.

- Stick to **larger strips** (instead of small pieces) at first.

- Avoid **sticky foods** (like nut butters alone) or **hard raw veggies**.

- Always **supervise meals and keep baby seated upright**.

Step 4: Gradual Expansion & Listening to Baby's Cues

Once your baby is comfortable, you can:
🦴 Introduce **more variety of meats and vegetables**.
🦴 Incorporate **fermented foods or dairy like kefir, yogurt, and cottage cheese** for probiotics.
🦴 Keep **avoiding grains, refined sugars, and processed foods** to support gut health.

- Encourage **eating with the family** to make mealtimes enjoyable.

Step 1: Prepare the Groundwork

Before you introduce solids, set yourself up for success with these key principles:

- **Prioritize high-quality ingredients.** Try to choose **grass-fed, pasture-raised, and organic** animal products whenever available. These contain more essential fatty acids, fat-soluble vitamins, and fewer toxins compared to conventional meats and dairy.

- **No added salt or sugar.** Babies' kidneys are still developing, and their taste buds are highly sensitive. Avoid processed foods, added sweeteners, and excessive salt.

- **Continue breastfeeding or formula feeding.** Solids complement, but do not replace, breastmilk or formula at this stage. These should remain the primary source of nutrition until at least 12 months, though breastfeeding is recommended for 24 months of age.

Once you have high-quality ingredients ready, it's time to start feeding!

Step 2: Begin with Chicken Stock for Digestive Support

The first food to introduce should be a gentle, gut-healing **chicken stock**. This nutrient-rich liquid provides essential amino acids, collagen, and minerals that help prepare the digestive system for solid foods.

How to Serve It:

- Offer **1-2 teaspoons** of warm stock in a small cup or spoon or before meals.

- Mix it into homemade purees for added nutrition.

- Chill in the refrigerator to change to a "jelly" that can be spoon fed or given for your little one to self feed.

Chicken stock acts as a gentle introduction to solids while supporting gut lining integrity and digestion.

Step 3: Introduce Soft, Nutrient-Dense Animal Fats

Next, incorporate **healthy, bioavailable fats** that mimic the nutrient profile of breastmilk. These include:

- **Grass-fed butter** – Rich in vitamin A, D, E and K2.

- **Ghee** – A lactose-free option that is easy to digest.

How to Serve It:

- Let your little one **lick a small amount** from a clean spoon or finger. You can give easy to grasp pieces for babies to feed themselves.

- Melt into chicken stock or mix into homemade purees.

- Use as a cooking fat for later foods (like egg yolks).

Animal fats **aid digestion, regulate blood sugar, and fuel brain development**—making them a perfect first food.

Step 4: Add in Bone Marrow & Meat (Purees or BLW)

Once your baby has tolerated fat, begin adding **bone marrow and pureed meats** for iron, protein, and critical vitamins.

How to Serve:

- **Roast marrow bones** and scoop out the soft, buttery marrow. Serve as is or mix under a whipped, buttery consistency has been formed. Offer small spoonfuls or blend into purees.

- **Pureed Meats:** Blend **grass-fed beef, lamb, or chicken** with a bit of **bone broth/stock, marrow, or breastmilk** for a soft, digestible consistency.

- **BLW (Baby-Led Weaning) Option:** Offer **soft-cooked meat strips** (like slow-cooked shredded beef or lamb) for baby to self-feed. Even by holding a piece of steak and gnawing on it, your little one will be able to suck out the nutrients. Once able to grasp, offer chicken legs or meat off the bone.

⬣ By 6–7 months, the iron stores in your little one become depleted and babies need **heme iron and zinc**, which are best absorbed from red meat.

Step 5: Egg Yolks

Egg yolks are a perfect **next step** because they provide **choline, DHA, and essential vitamins** for brain development.

How to Serve:

- Use **pasture-raised eggs** for the highest nutrient content.

- Soft-boil or lightly scramble the **yolk only** (the white contains anti-nutrients that may be harder to digest).

- Cook in **grass-fed butter, tallow, or ghee** for extra fat-soluble vitamins.

- Offer a small spoonful or let the baby feed themselves.

Step 6: Gradual Variety—Adding More Nutrient-Dense Foods

Once your baby has tolerated these foundational foods, **slowly introduce variety** by incorporating other ancestral superfoods:

- **Sardines, salmon, and other wild caught fish (for BLW)** – A powerhouse of omega-3s, calcium, and vitamin D.

- **Whole milk yogurt, goat cheese, kefir, and cottage cheese** – Provide probiotics and essential fats for gut health.

- **Liver (1-2x per week)** – The most nutrient-dense organ meat, offering iron, vitamin A, and B12.

- **Slow-cooked meats** – Lamb, beef, and chicken in broth-based stews.

Introduce **one new food at a time**, allowing a few days to monitor for any reactions before moving on.

Step 7: Incorporate Vegetables Rich in Healthy Fats & Key Vitamins

By 7 months, start adding carefully selected **foods that complement the ancestral diet**, focusing on those high in **vitamins and minerals**

- **Carrots & winter squash** – Rich in beta-carotene.
- **Lentils, black beans, chickpeas** – loaded with vitamins and minerals.
- **Beets** – Support digestion and blood health.
- **Avocado** – A perfect first plant food due to its healthy fats.
- **Fermented vegetables** – Sauerkraut or kimchi (small amounts) for probiotics.
- **Mashed peas or green beans** are other easy vegetables to incorporate into meals

How to Serve:

- Mash with **butter, bone broth, or ghee** for better absorption.

- Offer small **steamed or sliced** pieces or more vegetable variety for BLW.

Month-by-Month Guide: Purees to BLW

- **Month 6** → Focus on **purees** with **chicken stock, fats (grass fed butter), and meats or whipped bone marrow.**

- **Month 7** → Begin **soft finger foods & baby-led weaning** with nutrient-dense options like **sardines, beans, slow-cooked meats, and egg yolks**.

- **Month 8+** → Continue increasing variety while keeping ancestral staples as the foundation.

By introducing these foods in **a structured, step-by-step approach**, you are ensuring your baby receives the most bioavailable nutrients in a way that supports digestion, metabolism, and long-term health.

This **7-step approach** ensures your baby gets the **best** possible start with solid foods—focusing on time-tested, nutrient-dense foods that have sustained human development for generations.

In the next chapter, we'll dive deeper into **meal ideas, preparation tips, and troubleshooting common feeding concerns** to make this process as simple and enjoyable as possible.

Chapter Five: Easy & Delicious Recipes for Every Stage

Introducing solid foods should be a joyful and nourishing experience for both you and your baby. By starting with simple, nutrient-dense recipes that align with the ancestral approach, you can ensure your baby is getting the best possible nourishment at every stage.

This chapter provides **easy, delicious recipes for each stage,** focusing on soft, digestible purees and gentle textures that support gut health and development.

Stage One: Purees & Soft Foods (6–8 Months)

These first foods should be soft, well-cooked, and easy to digest. You can prepare them in small batches and store leftovers in the fridge or freezer for convenience.

---

1. Nourishing Chicken Stock Baby Broth

A simple, nutrient-rich broth to introduce before solids or mix into purees.

Ingredients:
- 1 whole pasture-raised chicken (or chicken feet for extra gelatin)
- 8 cups filtered water
- 1 tablespoon apple cider vinegar

Instructions:

1. Place the chicken in a pot and cover with filtered water.
2. Add apple cider vinegar and let sit for 30 minutes.
3. Bring to a gentle boil, then reduce to low and simmer for 6–12 hours.
4. Strain, cool, and serve small spoonfuls to your baby or mix into purees. Freeze for future use.

Serving Tip: Start with a teaspoon before meals to help digestion.

---

2. Creamy Egg Yolk Mash

Egg yolks are rich in **choline, DHA, and fat-soluble vitamins**, making them an ideal first food.

Ingredients:
- 1 pastured egg yolk
- 1 teaspoon grass-fed butter or ghee

Instructions:

1. Soft-boil the egg for **6 minutes** and remove the yolk.
2. Mash with warm butter or ghee for a smooth consistency.
3. Try spoon feeding or letting baby eat themselves

🥣 **Serving Tip:** Start with **half a yolk** before increasing the portion.

---

3. Bone Marrow & Beef Puree

A powerhouse of **iron, zinc, and brain-boosting fats**.

Ingredients:
- 2 marrow bones (roasted, marrow scooped out)
- ¼ cup grass-fed beef (cooked and tender)
- ¼ cup homemade bone broth

Instructions:

1. Roast marrow bones at 375°F (190°C) for **15–20 minutes**.

2. Scoop out marrow and blend with cooked beef and bone broth until smooth.

3. Serve warm, in small spoonfuls.

🥣 **Serving Tip:** Blend extra and freeze in small portions for later use.

---

4. Buttered Root Vegetable Mash

A gentle, digestible puree rich in **vitamin A and healthy fats**.

Ingredients:
 🦴 ½ cup cooked carrots, butternut squash, or sweet potato
 🦴 1 tablespoon grass-fed butter or ghee
 🦴 2 tablespoons chicken stock

Instructions:

1. Steam or roast vegetables until soft.

2. Mash with warm butter and chicken stock until smooth.

3. Serve warm.

🥣 **Serving Tip:** Avoid over-sweetening baby's palate by focusing on a balance of savory flavors.

---

5. Coconut Cream & Avocado Blend

A dairy-free, gut-friendly fat bomb packed with **healthy MCTs**.

Ingredients:
- ½ ripe avocado
- ¼ cup full-fat coconut cream

Instructions:

1. Mash or blend together until smooth.

2. Serve with a spoon or let baby self-feed with fingers.

🥣 **Serving Tip:** This makes a great introduction to **healthy plant-based fats**.

6. Slow-Cooked Lentil & Goat Cheese Puree

A **gentle protein source** with added probiotics.

Ingredients:
- ¼ cup soaked lentils
- ½ cup bone broth
- 1 teaspoon goat cheese

Instructions:

1. Soak lentils overnight to improve digestibility.
2. Simmer in bone broth until soft.
3. Blend with goat cheese until creamy.

🥣 **Serving Tip:** Lentils can be a great **complement** to an animal-based diet, but should not replace meats.

---

7. Simple Grass-Fed Meat Puree

A perfect iron-rich first meal for babies.

Ingredients:
- ½ cup cooked grass-fed beef, lamb, or chicken
- ¼ cup bone broth or breastmilk

Instructions:

1. Cook meat until very tender.
2. Blend with broth or breastmilk until smooth.
3. Serve warm.

🥣 **Serving Tip:** If doing **BLW**, offer shredded, slow-cooked meat instead.

Making Mealtime Enjoyable & Nutrient-Dense

- **Mix and Match** – Combine **buttered vegetables with egg yolks** or **meat purees with bone broth** to create new flavors.

- **Encourage Exploration** – Let your little one touch, smell, and taste a variety of textures.

- **Keep It Simple** – No need for complicated meals—focus on **whole, nourishing foods**.

Stage Two: Chunkier Textures & Finger Foods (8–10 Months)

At this stage, your baby is ready for more independence with food. The goal is to **move from smooth purees to mashed, soft foods and small finger foods.**

What to Introduce:

- **Mashed meats** (beef, lamb, chicken, or fish)
- **Bone marrow** (spread on sourdough or mashed into veggies)
- **Small pieces of soft-cooked vegetables**
- **Self-fed dairy** (whole milk yogurt, cottage cheese)
- **Sourdough bread** (gut-friendly alternative to conventional bread)
- **More BLW options** (soft-cooked steak strips, chicken drumsticks, lamb chops)
- **Sardines** (soft, omega-3-rich fish for easy chewing)

---

1. Mashed Beef & Bone Marrow Bowl

A delicious, nutrient-packed dish perfect for iron and brain development.

Ingredients:
- ¼ cup slow-cooked beef (grass-fed)

- 1 teaspoon roasted bone marrow
- 1 tablespoon bone broth

Instructions:

1. Mash the **beef and bone marrow** together with a fork.
2. Add **bone broth** to soften if needed.
3. Let baby self-feed using a spoon or eat with hands.

Tip: Serve with a soft-boiled egg yolk for extra choline and DHA.

---

2. Soft Roasted Vegetables with Butter

Perfect for little hands to grab and chew.

Ingredients:
- Carrots, squash, beets, or zucchini
- 1 tablespoon **grass-fed butter**

Instructions:

1. Slice vegetables into **finger-sized pieces**.

2. Roast at 375°F (190°C) for **20 minutes**, until very soft.

3. Toss with **melted butter** and serve warm.

🥣 **Tip:** These are great for practicing chewing while providing key vitamins like **A and C**.

---

3. Sourdough Bread with Liver Pâté

A great way to introduce iron-rich **organ meats**, but should only be given **1–2 times per week**.

Ingredients:
- 1 slice **sourdough bread**
- 1 teaspoon **homemade liver pâté**

Instructions:

1. Spread a **thin layer** of pâté on warm sourdough.

2. Cut into strips for easy grabbing.

🥣 **Tip:** Liver is a powerhouse of **iron, B vitamins, and vitamin A**, but should be limited due to its high vitamin A content.

---

4. Self-Feed Yogurt or Cottage Cheese

Supports gut health with **probiotics and healthy fats**.

Ingredients:
- ¼ cup full-fat **plain yogurt**
- 1 tablespoon **cottage cheese**

Instructions:

1. Let baby scoop with fingers or use a pre-loaded spoon.
2. Serve with **soft fruit or vegetables** (like mashed banana) if tolerated.

Tip: Opt for **raw or grass-fed dairy** for the best nutrient profile.

---

5. Sardines with Butter (Baby-Led Weaning Style)

Sardines are **rich in omega-3s and calcium**, making them a perfect finger food.

Ingredients:
- 1 small, boneless sardine (in water)
- ½ teaspoon grass-fed **butter**

Instructions:

1. Mash the sardine lightly with **butter**.
2. Offer in **small pieces** or full sardine for baby to self feed.

🥣 **Tip:** This is a great way to introduce seafood early for brain development.

Stage Three: More Textures & Family Foods (10–12 Months)

By this stage, babies can start **eating what the family eats**, with some modifications. The focus should be on **roasted meats, stews, soft-cooked vegetables, and more variety**.

What to Introduce:

🦴 **More whole meats** (small pieces of steak, shredded lamb, chicken drumsticks)
🦴 **Family meals** (fish, roasted meats, pasta, vegetable sides)
🦴 **More vegetables** (begin to expand variety)
🦴 **Fruits (closer to 1 year)** to maintain balanced sugar intake

1. Family Stew with Bone Broth

A **one-pot meal** rich in minerals and protein.

Ingredients:
- 1 lb **grass-fed beef or lamb** (stew meat)
- 4 cups **bone broth**
- 1 cup soft vegetables (carrots, squash, zucchini)
- 1 teaspoon **butter or ghee**

Instructions:

1. Slow-cook **meat and vegetables** in **bone broth** for 3–4 hours.

2. Serve small, soft pieces for baby while the family enjoys the full stew.

Tip: This makes mealtimes easier, as baby can eat with the rest of the family. Another nutrient dense food that can be sourced by your local butcher- beef tongue!

---

2. Small Pieces of Steak or Chicken Legs

Great for chewing practice and self-feeding.

Ingredients:
🦴 Grass-fed **steak, lamb chop, or chicken drumstick**

Instructions:

1. Cook steak and slice into **thin strips**.
2. Slow-cook **chicken drumsticks** until the meat falls off the bone.
3. Let baby **gnaw on the bone** for extra minerals!

🥣 Tip: Helps develop **jaw strength and chewing coordination**.

Snack Ideas for All Stages

🦴 **Bone broth popsicles** – Freeze homemade **bone broth** for a refreshing, mineral-rich snack.
🦴 **Avocado & butter mash** – Mix together for a creamy, healthy-fat snack.
🦴 **Sourdough toast with ghee** – A gut-friendly carb option with beneficial fats.
🦴 **Porridge with bone broth** – Use **lentils or soaked oats** with broth for extra minerals.
🦴 **Cottage cheese.**

Transitioning to More Fruits & Vegetables Closer to 1 Year

While **animal-based nutrition** remains the foundation, **expanding plant variety** is important for **gut health and fiber intake**.

You can opt to start incorporating the following once you have established a strong ancestral base:
  🦴 **More vegetables** – Spinach, beets, cauliflower, etc.
  🦴 **Fruits (in moderation)** – Berries, apples, citrus for vitamin C.
  🦴 **Herbs & spices** – Basil, turmeric, cinnamon for added nutrients.

Encouraging Family Foods & Minimizing Separate Meals

As baby moves toward **12 months and beyond**, aim to:

- Serve the same **stews, roasts, and slow-cooked meats** as the family.

- Avoid making separate "baby meals"—just modify textures.

- Offer **ancestral, whole foods** instead of processed snacks.

Chapter Six: Addressing Concerns & Challenges

Starting your baby on an ancestral diet is one of the best decisions you can make for their long-term health. However, like any journey, there may be challenges along the way. From food allergies to sourcing high-quality ingredients and handling picky eating, this chapter will guide you through potential obstacles with **practical solutions** to keep your baby on the path of optimal nutrition.

---

1. Understanding & Preventing Allergies

One of the biggest concerns when introducing solids is the risk of food allergies. Research now shows that **delayed introduction of allergenic foods** may actually increase the likelihood of developing allergies.

Why Ancestral Foods May Reduce Allergies

An ancestral approach supports gut health, which plays a **key role in immune system development**. Traditional foods like **bone broth, animal fats, and**

fermented dairy help strengthen the gut lining, making it more resilient to allergens.

Top Allergenic Foods to Introduce Carefully

- **Eggs** (especially egg whites)
- **Dairy** (cheese, yogurt, kefir—preferably raw or fermented)
- **Fish & Shellfish** (sardines, salmon, shrimp)
- **Nuts & Seeds** (nut butters, tahini)

How to Safely Introduce Allergens

🦴 **Start small** – Offer a tiny amount and wait **3–5 days** before increasing the portion.
🦴 **Pair with gut-supportive foods** – Introduce allergens alongside **bone broth, fats, or probiotics** to support digestion.
🦴 **Watch for reactions** – Symptoms like rashes, vomiting, or digestive upset may indicate an intolerance.

🥣 **Tip:** If your family has a history of allergies, consult a professional before introducing high-risk foods.

🥣 **Tip:** Adding sauerkraut brine to foods to aid in gut health

2. Overcoming Taste Preferences & Food Refusals

Some babies take to an ancestral diet immediately, while others may need **more exposure** to develop a taste for nutrient-dense foods like liver, marrow, and fermented dairy.

Understanding Taste Development

Babies are naturally inclined to prefer **sweet flavors**, which is why it's important to introduce **savory and umami-rich foods first**—before they become too accustomed to fruit or carbs.

Strategies to Encourage Acceptance

- **Repeat exposure** – It can take **8–10 tries** for a baby to accept a new food. Keep offering it!
- **Mix with familiar flavors** – Blend liver with beef, or mix egg yolk with bone broth.
- **Change the texture** – If your baby refuses mashed liver, try spreading pâté on sourdough instead.

🍖 **Tip:** Avoid **rewarding with sweet foods** (e.g., "eat your meat and you'll get fruit"). This teaches babies to crave sweets rather than appreciating nutrient-dense foods.

3. Sourcing High-Quality Ingredients

Finding **grass-fed, organic, and nutrient-dense foods** is crucial for the ancestral diet, but it can be **challenging or expensive** depending on where you live.

Best Sources for High-Quality Foods

- **Local Farmers & Butchers** – Seek out **grass-fed meats, raw dairy, and fresh eggs**.

- **Farmer's Markets** – Great for **organic produce, pasture-raised eggs, and raw cheeses**.

- **Online Meat Suppliers** – Companies like **White Oak Pastures, US Wellness Meats, and local co-ops** offer shipping.

- **Buying in Bulk** – Purchase **whole animals, bulk marrow bones, or frozen organ meats** to save money.

🥣 **Tip:** Prioritize **animal products** first (meats, fats, and dairy), then fill in with **seasonal produce and fermented foods**.

4. Handling Picky Eaters

As babies become toddlers, **picky eating** can develop due to growth spurts, teething, or asserting independence. However, picky eating is often **a learned behavior**, influenced by **processed foods, excess snacking, and parental pressure**.

Preventing & Managing Picky Eating

🦴**Set a good example** – Babies mimic what they see! If they see you enjoying steak and buttered veggies, they're more likely to eat them too.
🦴 **Stick to real food** – Avoid filling up on processed snacks, crackers, or sweetened foods.
🦴**Make food fun** – Offer foods in different forms (e.g., beef meatballs instead of a plain steak).
🦴 **Don't pressure or bribe** – Keep meals relaxed. Serve the food, and if they don't eat, they'll try again at the next meal.

🥣 **Tip:** Hunger is the best motivator—**avoid constant snacking**, and your child will be more willing to eat at mealtime.

5. Balancing Convenience & Ancestral Eating

Many parents worry that ancestral eating **requires too much cooking**, but with some planning, it can be just as simple as any other approach.

Meal Prep Tips for Busy Parents

🦴 **Batch cook** – Make **large batches** of broth, stews, and slow-cooked meats to last all week.
🦴 **Keep it simple** – Meals don't need to be fancy—**grass-fed ground beef, buttered veggies, and sourdough** make an easy dinner.
🦴 **Use leftovers** – Cook extra steak or roasted chicken so you have quick meals for the next day.

🥣 **Tip:** Ancestral eating doesn't mean spending hours in the kitchen—it's about choosing **whole, nutrient-dense ingredients** over processed foods.

Chapter Seven: Making Ancestral Eating a Lifestyle

1. Creating a Family Culture of Nutrient-Dense Eating

The best way to ensure **long-term health** for your child is to **create an environment where real food is the norm**. Babies and toddlers learn by **watching, mimicking, and participating**—so the way the whole family eats **shapes their habits for life**.

Why This Matters

🦴 Babies and children **copy what they see**—if they see you enjoying real food, they will too.
🦴 Processed foods **hijack taste preferences**, making it harder to appreciate real food.
🦴 A culture of whole, traditional foods **creates a positive food relationship** for life.

How to Make It Easy

Eat together as a family – Meals should be a shared experience, not separate "kid meals" vs. "adult meals."

Keep only real food in the house – If processed snacks aren't available, they won't be an option.
Make food preparation enjoyable – Involve your child in cooking, even at a young age.
Avoid labeling foods as "good" or "bad" – Instead, teach that **real food nourishes and fuels the body**.

🥣 **Tip:** If a child grows up eating **real, nutrient-dense foods**, they won't crave processed junk—because their body is getting what it truly needs!

---

2. Supporting Baby's Development Beyond Solids

Your baby's nutrition doesn't stop with solids. Beyond food, their overall development is **deeply influenced by lifestyle factors** that support gut health, brain function, and physical well-being.

Key Areas of Development

Sunlight & Outdoor Play – Supports vitamin D production, strong bones, and immune health.
Movement & Physical Activity – Crawling, walking, and exploring strengthen neural pathways.
Minimizing Toxins – Avoid processed foods, seed oils, and unnecessary additives.
Adequate Sleep – Critical for brain growth and

hormonal balance.
Connection & Stress Reduction – Babies thrive on loving, secure environments.

🥣 **Tip:** Nutrition is **one piece of the puzzle**—but lifestyle habits like **play, fresh air, and movement** are just as important!

---

3. Sustainable Eating for Families

Eating ancestrally isn't just beneficial for your baby—it's also better for the **environment, local farmers, and ethical food systems**.

How to Eat More Sustainably

Prioritize grass-fed and pasture-raised meats – This supports small farms and healthier ecosystems.
Buy local and seasonal – Farmer's markets and co-ops offer the freshest, most nutrient-dense foods.
Reduce food waste – Use bone broth, scraps, and leftovers creatively.
Teach children where food comes from – Involve them in gardening, visiting farms, or even small-scale homesteading.

🥣 **Tip:** Ethical eating isn't just about food—it's about **respecting nature, animals, and the health of future generations.**

4. How to Feed Your Baby After One Year

After **12 months**, your baby transitions into a toddler, and their diet naturally expands. The focus remains on **nutrient density**, but variety and mealtime independence also increase.

What Changes After One?

More family foods – Baby can now eat **what the family eats**, with minimal modification.
More texture and chewing practice – Move from soft textures to **more fibrous and chewy foods**.
More balanced meals – Protein, healthy fats, and fiber should be the foundation.
Gradual fruit introduction – Low-sugar fruits like **berries, citrus, and cooked apples** are ideal.

What to Keep Prioritizing

- Bone broths & nutrient-dense soups
- Grass-fed meats, organ meats, and seafood
- Raw and fermented dairy (yogurt, kefir, cheese)
- Butter, ghee, and tallow for brain and gut health
- Homemade snacks and whole foods over processed baby snacks

🥣 **Tip: The goal is not to transition to "kid food" but to continue prioritizing whole, nourishing meals.**

---

5. Keeping It Simple: Practical Tips for Everyday Life

Sticking to an ancestral diet **doesn't have to be complicated**. By keeping a **few simple habits in place**, nutrient-dense eating becomes effortless.

🦴 **Stock your kitchen with whole foods** – If you have real food available, making healthy meals is easy.
🦴 **Stick to simple meals** – Roasted meats, buttered veggies, fermented dairy—it doesn't have to be gourmet!
🦴 **Meal prep basics** – Make broths, cook meats in bulk, and keep easy-to-grab foods on hand.
🦴 **Be flexible & realistic** – Life happens! Do your best but don't stress over perfection.

🥣 **Tip:** Eating ancestrally isn't about "rules"—it's about **nourishing your family in a way that works for your lifestyle.**

Sample Weekly Meal Plan for Babies Transitioning to Solids (6-12 Months)

This meal plan follows a **gradual introduction** of ancestral foods, focusing on **nutrient density, digestibility, and developmental needs**.

Week 1-2 (First Foods, 6 Months)

Morning: Chicken stock mixed with mashed egg yolk
Midday: Buttered mashed carrots or sweet potatoes
Dinner: Blended meat puree (slow-cooked beef or lamb in broth)

Week 3-4 (Expanding Nutrients, 6-7 Months)

Morning: Bone marrow mixed with egg yolk
Midday: Avocado mashed with grass-fed butter
Dinner: Pureed liver with bone broth & blended veggies

Month 2-3 (BLW & More Texture, 7-8 Months)

Morning: Soft-boiled egg yolk with ghee & mashed avocado
Midday: Small bites of slow-cooked meat or shredded chicken

Dinner: Salmon and sourdough + buttered steamed veggies

Month 4-5 (More Finger Foods, 9-10 Months)

Morning: Whole milk yogurt + mashed banana
Midday: Sardines + roasted squash with butter
Dinner: Small pieces of steak or lamb + fermented veggies

Months 6+ (Toddler Transition, 10-12 Months)

Morning: Scrambled eggs in butter + sauerkraut
Midday: Slow-cooked beef stew with marrow-rich broth
Dinner: Roasted chicken drumsticks + sautéed greens

Chapter 8: Essential Feeding Considerations for Safety and Success

1. Recognizing Adverse Food Reactions

   - **Signs of an Allergic Reaction:**

     - Hives, swelling (especially around the face, lips, or eyes)

     - Vomiting or diarrhea shortly after eating

     - Coughing, wheezing, or difficulty breathing (seek emergency help immediately)

     - Irritability, excessive crying, or signs of discomfort after eating

   - **Signs of Food Intolerances or Sensitivities:**

     - Frequent gas, bloating, or digestive discomfort

     - Eczema or skin rashes

- Changes in stool (mucus, diarrhea, constipation)
- Sleep disturbances

2. Choking vs. Gagging: What's Normal?

- **Gagging:** A natural reflex that helps prevent choking and is common as babies learn to eat.
- **Choking:** A serious emergency where food blocks the airway.
- **How to Minimize Choking Risks:**
  - Offer soft, appropriately sized pieces of food.
  - Avoid round, hard, or sticky foods (grapes, whole nuts, popcorn, large chunks of meat).
  - Always supervise mealtimes.
  - Learn infant CPR for emergency preparedness.

3. Foods to Avoid in the First Year

- **Honey** (risk of botulism)

- **Whole nuts and large chunks of tough meats** (choking hazard)

- **Processed foods and added sugars** (can disrupt gut and metabolic health)

- **Unpasteurized dairy or raw milk** (risk of bacterial infections)

- **Certain high-mercury fish** (like swordfish and shark)

4. Proper Seating and Positioning for Safe Eating

- Babies should always sit **upright** in a **properly supported high chair** with a **90-degree angle at the hips, knees, and ankles** to reduce the risk of choking.

- Avoid **reclined feeding positions** when introducing solids.

- Ensure the baby is **fully alert and engaged** during mealtimes.

5. Best Utensils for Early Eating

- **Soft-tipped spoons** for parent-led feeding and early self-feeding.

- **Open cups** (like small shot glass-sized training cups) to encourage proper drinking skills.

- **Silicone or stainless steel baby utensils and plates** for introducing self-feeding around 9-10 months.

Conclusion: Celebrating This Transition & The Power of Returning to Our Roots

By choosing an **ancestral, whole-food approach**, you are doing more than just feeding your baby…

- Your child will grow up **knowing what real food is**.

- They will **thrive on strong digestion, brain function, and immunity**.

- You will **break the cycle of processed, modern diets** that lead to chronic health issues.

This journey is about **more than just nutrition, it's about creating a lifestyle that supports optimal health for you, your child, and future generations.**

Introducing your baby to their **first foods** is more than just a milestone, it's a **celebration of nourishment, tradition, and a return to ancestral wisdom**. You have embarked on a journey that not only supports your child's **growth and development** but also strengthens their **gut health, brain function, and immune system** for years to come.

The Long-Term Benefits of Returning to Our Roots

- **Strong immune systems** – Babies raised on real, ancestral foods are less prone to chronic illness and inflammation.

- **Better digestion & gut health** – A strong microbiome leads to fewer allergies, sensitivities, and digestive issues.

- **Optimal brain development** – Nutrients like choline, DHA, and fat-soluble vitamins help build a strong, resilient brain.

- **A love for real food** – By starting with savory, nutrient-dense foods, your baby will develop a preference for wholesome meals.

- **Lifelong health** – Avoiding ultra-processed, sugar-laden foods helps prevent metabolic disorders and lifestyle diseases later in life.

Appendix

Glossary of Common Terms in Ancestral Nutrition

Nutrients & Their Roles

- **DHA (Docosahexaenoic Acid)** – An essential omega-3 fatty acid crucial for **brain and eye development**. Found in wild-caught fish, grass-fed meats, and pastured egg yolks.

- **Choline** – A vital nutrient for **brain function and memory development**. Found in egg yolks, liver, and grass-fed dairy.

- **Collagen & Gelatin** – Supports gut health, joint development, and skin integrity. Found in **bone broth and slow-cooked meats**.

- **Fat-Soluble Vitamins (A, D, E, K2)** – Critical for **immune function, bone growth, and neurological health**. Found in **butter, egg yolks, liver, and animal fats**.

- **Probiotics & Fermented Foods** – Promote a **healthy gut microbiome**, reducing the risk of allergies and digestive issues. Found in **kefir,**

yogurt, and sauerkraut.

Key Ancestral Foods

- **Bone Broth** – Rich in minerals and amino acids that support gut health, immunity, and digestion.

- **Grass-Fed Butter & Ghee** – Provides essential fats and fat-soluble vitamins for brain and hormonal development.

- **Organ Meats (Liver, Heart, Kidney)** – Some of the most nutrient-dense foods on earth, packed with iron, B vitamins, and choline.

- **Fermented Dairy (Kefir, Yogurt, Raw Cheese)** – Supports digestion and delivers beneficial probiotics.

- **Pasture-Raised Eggs** – A perfect first food, high in choline, healthy fats, and essential vitamins.

- **Wild-Caught Fatty Fish (Sardines, Salmon, Mackerel)** – A powerhouse of DHA and omega-3s.

Resources for Sourcing High-Quality Ingredients

Where to Buy Grass-Fed Meats, Organ Meats, and Bone Broth Ingredients

- **White Oak Pastures** – A trusted source for **grass-fed meats, pasture-raised poultry, and organ meats**.

- **US Wellness Meats** – Offers **bulk options** for nutrient-dense meats, bones, and fats.

- **Local Farmers & Co-Ops** – Visit **farmer's markets** or find **a local CSA** (community-supported agriculture).

Best Places to Find Pasture-Raised Dairy & Fermented Foods

- **Local raw dairy farms** – Check www.realmilk.com to find farms near you.

- **Organic, grass-fed yogurt & kefir** – Look for brands that prioritize **fermented, full-fat dairy**.

Best Sources for Wild-Caught Fish

- **Vital Choice Seafood** – A great source for **wild salmon, sardines, and mackerel**.

- **Local fish markets** – Buy **fresh, wild-caught options** whenever possible.

"Introducing Solid Foods for Babies." *Better Health Channel*, State Government of Victoria, https://www.betterhealth.vic.gov.au/health/healthyliving/eating-tips-for-babies.

"How Long Should You Breastfeed? Here's What Experts Say." *GoodRx Health*, https://www.goodrx.com/health-topic/pregnancy/breastfeeding-guidelines.

"Consequences of Incomplete Carbohydrate Absorption from Fruit Juice Consumption in Infants." *PubMed*, https://pubmed.ncbi.nlm.nih.gov/8571325/.

"Why Ditch the Infant Cereals?" *Food Renegade*, https://www.foodrenegade.com/why-ditch-infant-cereals/

"BASICS." *Food Renegade*, https://www.foodrenegade.com/basics/.

"Why We're Bringing Back These 6 Traditional First Foods for Babies." *Noelle's Naturals*, https://noellesnaturals.com/blogs/news/why-we-re-bringing-back-these-6-traditional-first-foods-for-babies.

"Baby Food Sold at Target Recalled Because of Lead Contamination." *Food Safety News*, https://www.foodsafetynews.com/2023/12/baby-food-sold-at-target-recalled-because-of-lead-contamination/.

"Why You Shouldn't Eat Enriched or Fortified Foods." *Deliciously Organic*, https://deliciouslyorganic.net/why-you-shouldnt-eat-enriched-or-fortified-foods/.

"Baby Food Around the World: What Baby's First Foods Are." *Amara Organic Foods*, https://amaraorganicfoods.com/blogs/blog/baby-food-around-the-world.

"Components of Human Breast Milk: From Macronutrient to Microbiome and microRNA." *PMC*, https://www.ncbi.nlm.nih.gov/pmc/articles/PMC7267092/.

"Baby Brain Food: 7 Foods to Fuel Brain Development." *UCLA Health*, https://www.uclahealth.org/news/baby-brain-food-7-foods-to-fuel-brain-development.

"Native Foods and Practices Supporting Infant Brain Development." *SpringerLink*, https://link.springer.com/article/10.1007/s10995-019-02745-4.

Printed in Dunstable, United Kingdom